DIABETIC GASTROPARESIS DIET COOKBOOK

Healthy Delicious Low-Carb, Low-Fiber Recipes to Manage Symptoms & Soothe Abdominal Pain.

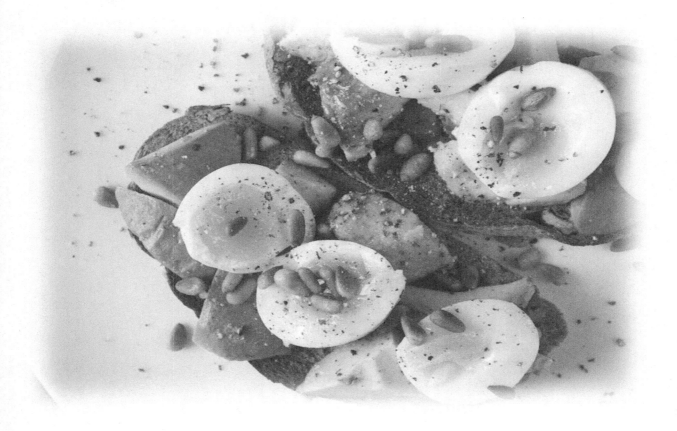

Christiana White

GAIN ACCESS TO MORE BOOKS

DISCLAIMER

The recipes in this cookbook are provided for informational purposes only and are not intended as medical or professional advice. While the author and publisher have made every effort to ensure the accuracy and effectiveness of the recipes, they are not responsible for any adverse effects r consequences resulting from the use of the suggestions herein.

The information in this cookbook should not replace professional advice. Readers are advised to consult a healthcare provider or a culinary professional before making any significant changes to their diet or cooking practices.

Nutritional information is approximate and should be used as a guide only. Variations may occur due to product availability, food preparation, portion size, and other factors.

The author and publisher disclaim any liability in connection with the use of this information. It is the reader's responsibility to determine the value and quality of any recipe or instructions provided for food preparation and to determine the nutritional adequacy of the food to be consumed.

ABOUT THE AUTHOR

When it comes to tasty and nutritious cookbooks that turn wellness into a delightful journey, Christiana White is the author you turn to. She approaches cooking from a new angle and has a passion for creating wholesome food.

Motivated by her own pursuit of health, Christiana's books on Amazon are brimming with delectable recipes that demonstrate that eating healthily can be both simple and enjoyable. Her creative method makes cooking approachable to all skill levels by fusing entire, simple foods with flavors from around the world.

Readers of Christiana's meals gush about the beneficial effects her foods have on their lives outside of the kitchen. Her books are more than just recipes; they're guides for a happier, better way of life, resulting in everything from more energy to a revitalized passion for cooking.

Come along with Christiana to discover how to turn your meals into satisfying and joyful experiences. Discover the delightful intersection of health and flavor by delving into the colourful world of her cookbooks.

TABLE OF CONTENTS.

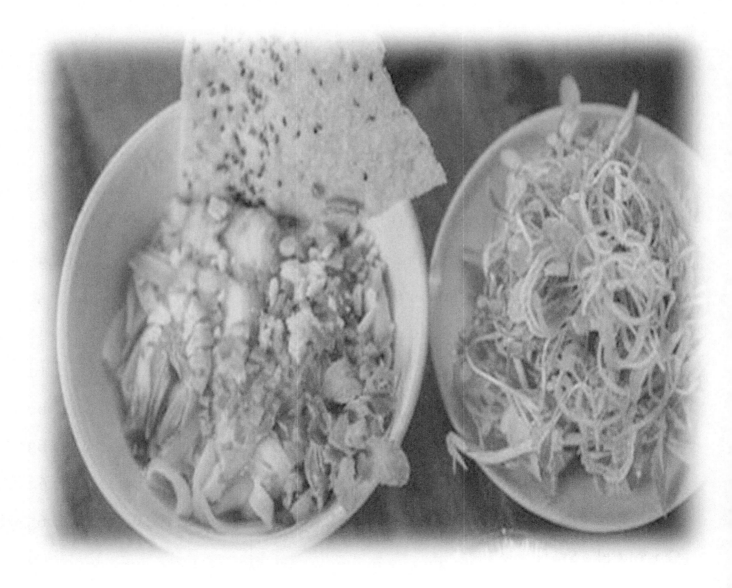

INTRODUCTION

A re you tired of being limited by diabetic gastroparesis? Do dull, uninteresting meals make you feel irritated and deprived? If so, this cookbook is your ticket to the gastronomic revolution.

As a nutritionist, I am aware of the special issues associated with diabetic gastroparesis. I've experienced firsthand how the appropriate foods may not only alleviate symptoms but also reignite your love of food. This cookbook is more than simply recipes; it's a thorough guide to changing your relationship with food and rediscovering your enjoyment of eating.

What Sets This Cookbook Apart

- **Expertly Crafted Recipes:** Each meal has been deliberately developed to be delicious, nutritious, and easy on the digestive system. Say goodbye to blandness and hello to bold flavors and sensations.
- **Empowering Knowledge:** This book contains more than just recipes. You'll obtain a thorough understanding of the diabetic gastroparesis diet, learn how to navigate restaurants, and discover meal planning and grocery shopping techniques.
- **Personalized Support:** We understand that everyone's experience is unique. That is why we have provided a 30-day food plan that may be customized to your specific needs and interests. To make things easier for you, we've added supplementary materials such as a detailed grocery shopping list and meal planning guide.

- **A Focus on Flavor:** We think that controlling a medical condition should not entail giving up the enjoyment of eating. That is why we have prioritized flavor in each dish. Prepare to rediscover the pleasure of food!

Who This Cookbook Is For?

- People with diabetic gastroparesis: Whether you were recently diagnosed or have been dealing with this ailment for years, this cookbook is a reliable companion on your culinary journey.
- Caregivers and Family Members: If you're cooking for someone with diabetic gastroparesis, this book will provide you with the information and recipes you need to prepare nutritious and enjoyable meals.
- Anyone looking for a healthier lifestyle: Even if you don't have diabetic gastroparesis, the recipes in this book are ideal for anybody wishing to focus gut health while eating flavourful, nutritious meals.

Turn the page and go on a gastronomic trip that will change your life. This cookbook is more than just recipes; it is about empowerment, education, and reclaiming the pleasure of eating. You deserve to relish each bite, and this cookbook will teach you how.

CHAPTER ONE

Understanding Diabetic Gastroparesis.

Diabetic gastroparesis is a diabetes-related illness characterized by a delayed emptying of the stomach's contents. This disorder has a substantial impact on one's quality of life, resulting in a variety of symptoms and problems that must be carefully managed.

What is Diabetic Gastroparesis?

Gastroparesis, also called delayed gastric emptying, is a condition in which the stomach takes too long to empty its contents. Diabetes is frequently caused by injury to the vagus nerve, which is responsible for telling the stomach muscles to contract and force food through the digestive system. High blood sugar levels over time can cause nerve damage, affecting the digestion process.

Symptoms & Complications

Diabetic gastroparesis symptoms can vary, but frequent ones include:

- Nausea, vomiting.
- Bloating and stomach discomfort.
- Heartburn or esophageal reflux
- Feeling full immediately after eating.
- Reduced appetite and weight loss

Diabetic gastroparesis can cause major complications, such as:

- Hypoglycaemia (low blood sugar) resulting from delayed food digestion and absorption.

- Diabetic ketoacidosis is a life-threatening disorder caused by the accumulation of acids in the blood.
- Malnutrition and vitamin deficits.
- Formation of bezoars, which are hardened, undigested foods that can clog the gastrointestinal track.

Diagnoses and Treatments

Diabetic gastroparesis is diagnosed using a combination of symptom assessment and medical tests, which include:

- To see the digestive tract, use barium X-rays or beefsteak meals.
- Radioisotope gastric-emptying scans to determine the pace of digestion.
- Gastric manometry, which measures stomach muscular contractions.
- Upper endoscopy to inspect the stomach lining.

Treatment for diabetic gastroparesis focuses on blood sugar control and nutritional changes. Strategies can include:

- Eating smaller and more frequent meals.
- Selecting low-fiber, low-fat foods that are easier to digest.
- Using drugs to induce stomach muscle contractions or alleviate nausea
- In severe situations, use feeding tubes or intravenous nutrition.

Living with diabetic gastroparesis necessitates a multifaceted approach that involves dietary adjustments, medication, and lifestyle modifications. It is critical to collaborate with healthcare specialists to create a specific plan that addresses both diabetes and gastroparesis.

Understanding diabetic gastroparesis and its ramifications allows people to take proactive efforts to manage their symptoms and maintain their quality of life.

Education, support, and continuing treatment are critical components for successfully treating this complex condition.

Diet in Managing Your Health

Dietary factors play a critical role in diabetic gastroparesis. It is essential for treating both gastroparesis symptoms and diabetes-related blood glucose levels. A well-planned diet can help avoid or alleviate gastroparesis symptoms while also ensuring that you get enough nutrients, calories, and water, particularly if you are malnourished or dehydrated as a result of gastroparesis.

Diabetic gastroparesis impairs the regular action of muscles in your stomach, slowing or even stopping digestion and causing glucose levels to fluctuate unpredictably. This complicates diabetes management since the timing of stomach emptying influences how your body maintains blood sugar levels after meals.

The Plate Method

The Plate Method is an effective technique for regulating your nutrition with diabetic gastroparesis. This includes visually partitioning your plate to guarantee a balanced lunch.

- Half of the dish filled with low-carbohydrate, non-starchy veggies.
- One-quarter of the plate should contain lean protein.
- The remaining quarter contains carbs, especially from low-fiber sources.

It's vital to highlight that people with diabetic gastroparesis have quite different nutritional needs. What works for one individual may not work for others. Regular monitoring of blood glucose levels and symptoms, as well as constant consultation

13

with healthcare specialists, are required to adjust dietary options to your unique needs.

The Effects of Diet on Quality of Life

Making smart food choices can dramatically improve your quality of life. The appropriate diet can help you manage symptoms, maintain nutritional status, and eat a wider range of foods while keeping your diabetes under control.

Diet plays a diverse and individualized role in diabetic gastroparesis treatment. Finding the correct combination of nutrients, consistency, and timing is essential for supporting your digestive system and efficiently managing your diabetes. You can improve your health and well-being by carefully planning and following dietary recommendations.

CHAPTER TWO: DIETARY GUIDELINES

The Essentials of Diabetic Gastroparesis Diet

Diabetic gastroparesis necessitates a unique approach to nutrition. It is defined by the stomach's failure to empty correctly, which can be aggravated by diabetes. The diet for this illness focuses on promoting stomach emptying and controlling blood sugar.

Key Dietary Considerations:

- Meal Frequency and Size: Eating smaller, more frequent meals keeps the stomach from becoming overly full, which can aggravate gastroparesis symptoms. It also improves blood sugar regulation.

- Food Consistency: Soft, well-cooked foods are generally recommended for simpler digestion. Raw, fibrous fruits and vegetables may be difficult to digest and should be avoided.

- Nutrient Intake: Ensuring that you get adequate vitamins and minerals is critical, as gastroparesis can cause shortages. A multivitamin supplement may be necessary.

- Hydration: Adequate fluid intake is required to avoid dehydration, which is a significant problem for people with gastroparesis.

- Carbohydrate Management: Controlling carbohydrate consumption is critical for blood sugar regulation. Consistent carbohydrate distribution across meals can help to maintain blood glucose levels.

How to Use This Cookbook for Maximum Results

This cookbook is intended to supply you with dishes that meet the dietary requirements of diabetic gastroparesis. To get the best results:

Follow the recipes closely.

- The recipes are designed to be gastroparesis-friendly while simultaneously meeting diabetic criteria.

Understand "Why":

- Understanding the reasons for dietary choices can allow you to make more informed meal decisions and better manage your condition.

Customize When Necessary

- Feel free to modify the recipes based on your specific tolerance and nutritional needs, but always keep the fundamental ideas in mind.

Monitor Your Health:

- Monitor your blood sugar levels and gastroparesis symptoms to understand how different foods influence you.

By following these rules and using the recipes supplied, you can eat tasty meals that benefit your health and well-being.

Key Principles: Low Carbohydrate, Low Sugar, And Easy Digestion.

The diet's basic concepts for managing diabetic gastroparesis are to decrease symptoms while maintaining stable blood glucose levels. Here's how these principles apply to daily eating habits:

Low Carb: Carbohydrates directly affect blood sugar levels. A low-carbohydrate diet helps to reduce these levels and effectively manage diabetes. It's recommended to choose complex carbs that have a lower glycemic index and give continuous energy without raising blood sugar levels.

Low Sugar: Sugar, particularly processed sugar, can induce rapid blood sugar spikes. To avoid these spikes and the difficulties that come with them, diabetic gastroparesis patients must limit their sugar consumption.

Foods that are easier to digest are vital for persons with gastroparesis because the condition causes the stomach to empty slowly. Soft, well-cooked, low-fiber foods can help avoid nausea and bloating.

Foods To Embrace and Avoid

Foods to embrace:

- Eggs are high in protein and easy to digest when prepared properly.
- Smooth peanut butter: Provides protein and fat without the fiber found in whole nuts.
- Banana: A low-fiber fruit that is easy on the stomach.
- White breads and refined cereals are lower in fiber and simpler to digest than whole grains.
- Cooked vegetables, such as zucchini, are easier to digest than uncooked ones.

Foods To Avoid:

- High-Fiber Foods: These include raw and dried fruits, as well as veggies like broccoli, which can create bezoars and blockages.
- Fatty Foods: Non-lean meats, as well as fried or fatty foods, can take longer to empty the stomach.
- Carbonated beverages may induce bloating and discomfort.
- Alcohol: Can impair blood sugar management and worsen gastroparesis symptoms.

Individuals with diabetic gastroparesis can enhance their overall quality of life by sticking to these dietary recommendations and making informed decisions about which foods to eat and which to avoid.

CHAPTER THREE: RECIPES

BREAKFAST RECIPES

Blueberry Smoothie

Serves: 1

Prep time: 5 minutes.

Ingredients:

- 1/2 cup of unsweetened almond milk.
- 1/2 cup blueberries, fresh or frozen.
- 1/4 cup plain Greek yogurt, non-fat
- One tablespoon of almond butter.
- One pinch of cinnamon (optional)

Instructions:

- Place all items in a blender.
- Blend until smooth.
- Serve immediately.

Nutritional value (estimated):

- Calories: 150.
- Carbohydrate: 18g
- Protein: 8 grams
- Fat: 7g
- Fiber: 4 grams.

Vegetable Omelet

Serves: 1

Prep time: 10 minutes.

Ingredients:

- Two big eggs.
- 1/4 cup chopped zucchini.
- 1/4 cup of chopped bell pepper.
- One tablespoon of chopped onion
- Non-stick cooking spray.

• Non-stick cooking spray.

- Add salt and pepper to taste.

Instructions:

- In a mixing basin, beat the eggs. Set aside.
- Cook the zucchini, bell pepper, and onion in a nonstick pan with cooking spray until soft.
- Pour the beaten eggs onto the vegetables.
- Cook until the eggs are set, then fold the omelet in half to serve.

Nutritional value (estimated):

- Calories:180
- Carbohydrate: 6g
- Protein: 12 grams
- Fat: 12g
- Fiber: 1 g.

Pumpkin Bisque

Servings: Two.

Prep time: 15 minutes.

Ingredients:

- One cup canned pumpkin puree.
- One cup of low-sodium vegetable broth
- 1/4 cup of light coconut milk.
- 1/2 tsp minced ginger.
- Add salt and pepper to taste.

Instructions:

- In a pot, blend the pumpkin puree and vegetable broth.
- Bring to a simmer, then add ginger.
- Cook for 5 minutes, then mix until smooth.
- Mix in the coconut milk, season with salt and pepper, and serve warm.

Nutritional value (estimated):

- Calories: 90.
- Carbs: 12g
- Protein: 2 grams
- Fat: 4g
- Fiber: 3 grams.

Egg Muffins

Servings: Six.

Prep time: 20 minutes.

Ingredients:

- Four big eggs.
- 1/4 cup diced cooked chicken breast.
- 1/4 cup chopped tomatoes; seeds removed.
- 1/4 cup shredded low-fat mozzarella cheese.
- Add salt and pepper to taste.

Instructions:

- Preheat the oven to 350°F/175°C.
- In a bowl, whisk together eggs, chicken, tomatoes, and cheese.
- Season with salt and pepper.
- Pour into muffin tins and bake for 15-20 minutes, or until firm.
- Allow to cool and serve.

Nutritional value (estimated):

- 100 calories per muffin.
- Carbs: 2g per muffin.
- Protein: 9 g per muffin.
- Fat: 6 g per muffin.
- Fiber: 0.5 g per muffin.

Cottage Cheese and Berries

Serves: 1

Prep time: 5 minutes.

Ingredients:

- 1/2 cup of low-fat cottage cheese
- 1/4 cup mixed berries (strawberries, raspberries, and blueberries).

Instructions:

- Put cottage cheese in a bowl.
- Garnish with mixed berries.
- Serve cold.

Nutritional value (estimated):

- Calories: 120.
- Carbohydrate: 10g
- Protein: 14 grams
- Fat: 2g
- Fiber: 2 grams.

Hard-boiled Eggs with Avocado

Serves: 1

Prep time: 10 minutes.

Ingredients:

- Two big eggs.
- One-half ripe avocado
- A pinch of salt.
- Ground black pepper (optional).

Instructions:

- Put eggs in a pot and cover with water. Bring to a boil, cover, and remove from the heat. Allow to sit for 8–10 minutes.
- Remove the eggs and place them in cold water to cool.
- Peel and cut the eggs in half.
- Slice the avocado and remove the pit. Scoop out the flesh and slice.
- Arrange the eggs and avocado on a plate. Season with salt and pepper to taste.

Nutritional value (estimated):

- Calories: 300.
- Carbs: 9g
- Protein: 15 grams.
- Fat: 23g
- Fiber: 7 grams.

Low-Fiber Cereal

Serves: 1

Prep time: 5 minutes.

Ingredients:

- One cup of low-fiber cereal (such as Rice Krispies or Corn Flakes).
- One cup almond milk or low-fat milk.

Instructions:

- Pour the cereal into a bowl.
- Add almond or low-fat milk.
- Stir and enjoy.

Nutritional value (estimated):

- Calories: 150.
- Carbohydrate: 30g
- Protein: 4 grams
- Fat: 2g
- Fiber: 1 g.

Banana Smoothie

Serves: 1

Prep time: 5 minutes.

Ingredients:

- Half ripe banana, frozen
- One cup unsweetened almond milk.
- One tablespoon of protein powder (optional)

Instructions:

- Place the frozen banana slices into a blender.
- If using, combine almond milk and protein powder.
- Blend until smooth.

Nutritional value (estimated):

- Calories: 120.
- Carbs: 19g
- Protein content: 2g (8g with protein powder).
- Fat: 4g
- Fiber: 3 grams.

Apple Slices with Nut Butter

Serves: 1

Prep time: 5 minutes.

Ingredients:

- One medium apple, peeled and sliced
- 1 tablespoon of smooth almond or peanut butter.

Instructions:

- Peel the apples and cut them into thin pieces.
- Spread almond or peanut butter on each slice.

Nutritional value (estimated):

- Calories:180
- Carbohydrate: 24g
- Protein: 4 grams
- Fat: 9g
- Fiber: 4 grams.

Cottage Cheese with Salted Almonds

Serves: 1

Prep time: 5 minutes.

Ingredients:

- 1/2 cup of low-fat cottage cheese
- 1 teaspoon salted almonds, diced

Instructions:

- Put cottage cheese in a bowl.
- Add chopped almonds on top.

Nutritional value (estimated):

- Calories: 120.
- Carbohydrate: 5g
- Protein: 15 grams.
- Fat: 5g
- Fiber: 0 grams

LUNCH RECIPES

Vegetable Soup

Servings: four.

Prep time: 15 minutes.

Ingredients:

- Two cups of vegetable broth (low sodium)
- 1 cup peeled and sliced carrots.
- 1 cup potatoes, peeled and diced
- 1/2 cup finely chopped spinach.
- Add salt and pepper to taste.

Instructions:

- In a large pot, heat the vegetable broth to a boil.
- Add carrots and potatoes, decrease heat, and cook until soft, about 10 minutes.
- Stir in the spinach and simmer for another 2 minutes.
- Season with salt and pepper and serve.

Nutritional Value per Serving:

- Calories: 80.
- Carbohydrate: 18g
- Fiber: 3 grams.
- Protein: 2 grams

Turkey Sandwich

Serves: 1

Prep time: 5 minutes.

Ingredients:

- Two slices of white bread
- 3 oz turkey breast, sliced
- lettuce
- 1 tablespoon mayonnaise (low fat)

Instructions:

- Spread mayonnaise onto one slice of bread.
- Add turkey breast and lettuce on top.
- Top with the second slice of bread, then cut in half.

Nutritional Value per Serving:

- Calories: 250.
- Carbohydrate: 25 grams
- Fiber: 1 g.
- Protein: 20 grams

Chicken and Goat Cheese Skillet

Servings: two.

Prep time: 20 minutes.

Ingredients:

- Two boneless, skinless chicken breasts.
- 1/4 cup crumbled goat cheese.
- One tablespoon of olive oil.
- Add salt and pepper to taste.

Instructions:

- Heat the olive oil in a skillet over medium heat.
- Season chicken breasts with salt and pepper, then cook until golden brown on both sides.
- Top each chicken breast with goat cheese and cover the skillet.
- Cook until the cheese is slightly melted and the chicken is fully cooked.

Nutritional Value per Serving:

- Calories: 300.
- Carbohydrate: 1g
- Fiber: 0 grams
- Protein: 30 grams

Curried Chicken Skillet.

Servings: four.

Prep time: 25 minutes.

Ingredients:

- Four boneless, skinless chicken thighs.
- One tablespoon of curry powder.
- 1 cup coconut milk (light)
- One tablespoon of olive oil.
- Salt to taste.

Instructions:

- Heat the olive oil in a skillet over medium heat.
- Season the chicken thighs with curry powder and salt.
- Cook the chicken until browned on both sides.
- Pour the coconut milk over the chicken and simmer until it is fully cooked.

Nutritional Value per Serving:

- Calories: 250.
- Carbs: 4g
- Fiber: 1 g.
- Protein: 20 grams

Pressure Cooker Pork Tacos

Servings: four.

Prep time: 30 minutes.

Ingredients:

- One-pound pork loin, sliced into strips
- One tablespoon of taco seasoning (low sodium)
- One-half cup water
- Eight tiny corn tortillas.
- One-half cup mango salsa

Instructions:

- Place the pork loin pieces into the pressure cooker.
- Season with taco seasoning and add water.
- Cook at high pressure for 20 minutes.
- Release the pressure and shred the pork with a fork.
- Serve on corn tortillas with mango salsa.

Nutritional Value per Serving:

- Calories: 300.
- Carbohydrate: 20g
- Fiber: 2 grams.
- Protein: 25 grams.

Chicken with Peach and Avocado Salsa

Servings: four.

Prep time: 20 minutes.

Ingredients:

- 4 boneless and skinless chicken breasts.
- One ripe peach, peeled and diced
- One ripe avocado, peeled and diced
- Juice from 1 lime
- Add salt and pepper to taste.

Instructions:

- Grill or bake the chicken breasts until well done.
- In a bowl, combine the peach, avocado, and lime juice.
- Season the salsa with salt and pepper.
- Top the chicken with the peach and avocado salsa.

Nutritional Value per Serving:

- Calories: 250.
- Carbohydrates: around 15g.
- Fiber: approximately 3g.
- Protein: around 30g.

Italian shrimp 'n' pasta

Servings: four.

Prep time: 30 minutes.

Ingredients:

- 8 ounces of pasta (choose a low-fiber kind).
- One-pound shrimp, peeled and deveined
- Two teaspoons of olive oil.
- 2 garlic cloves, minced
- 1 cup low sodium tomato sauce
- Fresh basil, chopped.
- Add salt and pepper to taste.

Instructions:

- Cook pasta according to package directions and drain.
- Heat olive oil in a skillet over medium heat. Cook shrimp until pink.
- Stir in the garlic and heat for another minute.
- Stir in the tomato sauce and cook for 5 minutes.
- Toss the pasta in the shrimp sauce and top with basil.
- Add salt and pepper to taste.

Nutritional Value per Serving:

- Calories: 350.
- Carbohydrates: around 45g.
- Fiber: approximately 2g.
- Protein: around 25g.

Tuna Teriyaki Kebabs

Servings: four.

Preparation time is 40 minutes (including marinating time).

Ingredients:

- Cut 1 pound tuna steak into cubes
- 1/4 cup of teriyaki sauce (low sodium)
- 1 bell pepper chopped into bits.
- 1 zucchini, sliced
- 1 onion sliced into wedges.

Instructions:

- Marinate the tuna cubes in teriyaki sauce for 30 minutes.
- Thread tuna and vegetables on skewers.
- Grill the tuna over medium heat until it reaches the desired doneness.

Nutritional Value per Serving:

- Calories: 200.
- Carbohydrates: around 10g.
- Fiber: approximately 2g.
- Protein: around 30g.

Milkshake

Servings: two.

Prep time: 10 minutes.

Ingredients:

- One ripe banana.
- One cup low-fat milk (or almond milk).
- One teaspoon of vanilla extract.
- Ice cubes (Optional)

Instructions:

- In a blender, mix the banana, milk, and vanilla essence.
- If desired, add ice cubes to create a thicker consistency.
- Blend until smooth.
- Serve in a chilled glass.

Nutritional Value per Serving:

- Calories: 150.
- Carbohydrates: around 30g.
- Fiber: approximately 3g.
- Protein: around 6g.

Applesauce

Servings: four.

Prep time: 10 minutes.

Cook for 30 minutes.

Ingredients:

- 4 medium apples (choose a low-sugar variety, such as Granny Smith.)
- 1/2 cup water.
- One teaspoon of ground cinnamon.
- 1/4 teaspoon ground nutmeg (optional).
- A squeeze of fresh lemon juice (optional).

Instructions:

- Peel, core, and cut apples into small pieces.
- In a saucepan over medium heat, combine the apples, water, and cinnamon.
- Cover and boil the apples for 25-30 minutes, or until tender.
- Once the apples have softened, use a potato masher or immersion blender to mash or blend them to the appropriate consistency.
- For a smoother texture, strain the applesauce using a fine mesh sieve.
- If preferred, add a squeeze of lemon juice for a tangy finish.
- Cool the applesauce before refrigerating. Serve cold.

Nutritional Value per Serving:

- Calories: around 95.
- Carbohydrates: About 25g.
- Fiber: approximately 4g.
- Protein: less than 1 gram.

DINNER RECIPES.

Baked Poultry or Fish

Servings: four.

Prep time: 10 minutes.

Cook time: 20 minutes.

Ingredients:

- 4 boneless, skinless chicken breasts or fish filets
- One tablespoon of olive oil.
- Add salt and pepper to taste.
- Lemon slices as garnish.

Instructions:

- Preheat your oven to 375°F (190°C).
- Place the chicken or fish into a roasting dish.
- Drizzle olive oil and season with salt and pepper.
- Bake for 20 minutes, or until a fork easily pierces the interior temperature of 165°F (74°C) in chicken or fish.
- Serve with lemon slices.

Nutritional Value per Serving:

- Calories: 165 (chicken); 145 (fish).
- Carbohydrate: 0g
- Fiber: 0 grams
- Protein: 25g (chicken) and 20g (fish).

Garlic Mashed Potatoes

Servings: four.

Prep time: 15 minutes.

Cook time: 20 minutes.

Ingredients:

- Two pounds of potatoes, peeled and cubed
- 4 garlic cloves, minced
- Half-cup low-fat milk
- Two tablespoons of unsalted butter.
- Salt to taste.

Instructions:

- Cook the potatoes and garlic in a pot of water until soft.
- Drain, then return to the pot.
- Combine milk and butter.
- Mash until smooth and creamy.
- Season with salt.

Nutritional Value per Serving:

- Calories: 200.
- Carbohydrate: 30g
- Fiber: 2 grams.
- Protein: 4 grams

Spinach And Cheese-Stuffed Chicken

Servings: four.

Prep time: 25 minutes.

Cook for 30 minutes.

Ingredients:

- Four chicken breasts.
- 1 cup spinach, boiled and drained.
- 1/2 cup of low-fat cream cheese
- 1/4 cup grated parmesan cheese.
- Add salt and pepper to taste.

Instructions:

- Preheat the oven to 350°F/175°C.
- Butterfly and flatten the chicken breasts.
- Combine spinach, cream cheese, and parmesan.
- Divide the mixture between the chicken breasts, roll them up, and secure with toothpicks.
- Bake for 30 minutes, or until the chicken is cooked through.

Nutritional Value per Serving:

- Calories: 300.
- Carbohydrate: 5g
- Fiber: 1 g.
- Protein: 30 grams

Fruit Cocktail

Servings: four.

Prep time: 10 minutes.

Ingredients:

- 1 cup canned peaches with no sugar added, drained
- 1 cup canned pears with no sugar added, drained
- 1 cup canned pineapple, no sugar added and drained
- 1/2 cup maraschino cherries with no sugar added

Instructions:

- In a bowl, combine all of the fruits.
- Chill in the fridge before serving.

Nutritional Value per Serving:

- Calories: 100.
- Carbohydrate: 25 grams
- Fiber: 2 grams.
- Protein: 1 gram.

Cilantro Bean Burgers

Servings: four.

Prep time: 15 minutes.

Cooking Time: 10 minutes.

Ingredients:

- One can (15 ounces) of black beans, drained and rinsed
- 1/4 cup chopped cilantro.
- 1/4 cup chopped onion.
- 1 egg
- One-half teaspoon cumin
- Add salt and pepper to taste.
- 1/4 cup breadcrumbs (gluten-free if desired)

Instructions:

- Mash the beans in a bowl.
- Combine the cilantro, onion, egg, cumin, salt, pepper, and breadcrumbs.
- Shape into patties and fry in a nonstick skillet over medium heat for 5 minutes per side.

Nutritional Value per Serving:

- Calories:180
- Carbohydrate: 30g
- Fiber: 6 grams.
- Protein: 10 grams.

Egg and Broccoli Slaw Wrap

Servings: two.

Prep time: 15 minutes.

Ingredients:

- Two big eggs.
- 1 cup broccoli slaw (pre-packaged and available at most grocery stores)
- Two low carb tortillas
- Add salt and pepper to taste.

Instructions:

- Cook the eggs in a nonstick pan over medium heat.
- Season the eggs with salt and pepper.
- Heat the tortillas in the microwave for 10 seconds.
- Spread half of the scrambled eggs and half of the broccoli slaw onto each tortilla.
- Roll the tortillas tightly to make wraps.

Nutritional Value per Serving:

- Calories: approximately 200.
- Carbohydrates: around 15g.
- Fiber: approximately 3g.
- Protein: around 12g.

Chicken with Low-Fat Crackers

Servings: four.

Prep time: 20 minutes.

Ingredients:

- 4 boneless and skinless chicken breasts.
- One tablespoon of olive oil.
- Add salt and pepper to taste.
- One box of low-fat crackers.

Instructions:

- Preheat your oven to 375°F (190°C).
- Season the chicken breasts with olive oil, salt, and pepper.
- Bake for 25 to 30 minutes, or until the chicken is thoroughly done.
- Serve the chicken with low-fat crackers as a side.

Nutritional Value per Serving:

- Calories: approximately 300.
- Carbohydrates: around 20g.
- Fiber: approximately 1g.
- Protein: around 30g.

Fruit Purees

Servings: four.

Prep time: 10 minutes.

Ingredients:

- Two cups mixed berries (strawberries, blueberries, raspberries)
- One ripe banana.
- One tablespoon of honey (optional)

Instructions:

- Using a blender, combine the mixed berries and banana until smooth.
- If you want it sweeter, add honey.
- Serve the purée cold.

Nutritional Value per Serving:

- Calories: around 100.
- Carbohydrates: around 25g.
- Fiber: approximately 4g.
- Protein: around 1g.

Vegetable Juice

Servings: two.

Prep time: 10 minutes.

Ingredients:

- Two carrots, peeled
- One tiny cucumber.
- 1 small beet, peeled
- 1/2 cup of spinach leaves.

Instructions:

- Wash all vegetables well.
- In a juicer, combine the carrots, cucumbers, beets, and spinach.
- Serve the juice immediately.

Nutritional Value per Serving:

- Calories: around 70.
- Carbohydrates: around 15g.
- Fiber: approximately 3g.
- Protein: around 2g.

SNACK AND DESSERT RECIPES

Plantain Chips

Servings: four.

Prep time: 10 minutes.

Cook for 15-18 minutes.

Ingredients:

- Two medium-green plantains.
- 2 teaspoons sunflower oil.
- 1/2 teaspoon garlic granules.
- 1/2 tsp black pepper.
- A pinch of cayenne pepper (optional).

Instructions:

- Preheat the oven to 190°C (170°C fan oven/gas 5).
- Peel the plantains and slice 1/8 inch thick.
- Add the oil, garlic granules, and black pepper.
- Spread in a single layer on a baking tray lined with nonstick paper.
- Bake for 15–18 minutes, or until thoroughly cooked and crisp.
- Allow to cool before topping with cayenne pepper, if desired.

Nutritional Value per Serving:

- Calories: around 200.
- Carbohydrates: around 27g.
- Fiber: approximately 8g.
- Protein: around 7g.

Sweet Potato Chips

Servings: four.

Prep time: 10 minutes.

Cook for 25-30 minutes.

Ingredients:

- Two huge sweet potatoes.
- One tablespoon olive oil.
- Salt to taste.

Instructions:

- Preheat your oven to 400°F (200°C).
- Thinly slice the sweet potatoes.
- Toss with olive oil and arrange in a single layer on a baking sheet.
- Bake for approximately 25-30 minutes, flipping halfway through.

Nutritional Value per Serving:

- Calories: around 150.
- Carbohydrates: around 35g.
- Fiber: around 5g.
- Protein: around 2g.

Peanut Butter Balls.

Serving size: 15 balls.

Prep time: 10 minutes.

Ingredients:

- 2/3 cup unsweetened peanut butter.
- 1/2 cup vanilla protein powder.
- 1/2 tablespoon chia seeds.
- 2 tablespoons unsweetened coconut flakes.
- One tablespoon of ground flax seed
- Stevia for taste.

Instructions:

- Blend together peanut butter, protein powder, chia seeds, flaxseed, coconut flakes, and stevia until smooth.
- Form the mixture into 1 to 1½-inch balls.
- Arrange on a dish and chill until firm.

Nutritional value per ball:

- Calories: around 130.
- Carbohydrates: around 7g.
- Fiber: approximately 2g.
- Protein: around 7g.

Roasted Chickpeas.

Servings: four.

Prep time: 5 minutes.

Cook for 25-30 minutes.

Ingredients:

- 1 can of chickpeas (400g)
- 2 teaspoons rapeseed oil.
- 1/2 teaspoon ground cumin.
- 1/2 teaspoon chili powder.

Instructions:

- Rinse, drain, and pat dry the chickpeas.
- Preheat the oven to 190°C (gas 5).
- Grease a baking tray and place in the oven for 3 minutes.
- Spread the chickpeas onto the tray and bake for 15 minutes.
- Toss with oil, cumin, and chili powder, and bake for an additional 10-15 minutes.

Nutritional Value per Serving:

- Calories: around 79.
- Carbohydrates: around 8g.
- Fiber: approximately 3g.
- Protein: around 4g.

Hummus

Servings: six.

Prep time: 10 minutes.

Ingredients:

- 1 can (400g) drained and washed chickpeas.
- One clove garlic
- Juice from 1 lemon
- One teaspoon of cayenne pepper.
- 4 tablespoons natural yogurt.
- Freshly ground black pepper.

Instructions:

- Combine all the ingredients in a food processor or blender.
- Blend until nearly smooth.
- Season to taste and serve.

Nutritional Value per Serving:

- Calories: around 59.
- Carbohydrates: around 7g.
- Fiber: approximately 2g.
- Protein: around 4g.

Guacamole

Servings: four.

Prep time: 10 minutes.

Ingredients:

- Two ripe avocados.
- Juice from 1 lime
- 2 tablespoons minced cilantro.
- Salt to taste.

Instructions:

- Halve the avocados, remove the pit, and scoop out the flesh into a basin.
- Using a fork, mash the avocado until it reaches the appropriate consistency.
- Stir in the lime juice, cilantro, and salt.
- Serve immediately or cover with plastic wrap and chill.

Nutritional Value per Serving:

- Calories: around 160.
- Carbohydrates: around 9g.
- Fiber: approximately 7g.
- Protein: around 2g.

Frozen Bananas

Servings: four.

Preparation time: 5 minutes (including freezing time)

Ingredients:

- Four ripe bananas.

Instructions:

- Peel the bananas and cut them into half-inch slices.
- Arrange the banana slices on a baking sheet coated with parchment paper.
- Freeze for 2-3 hours, until solid.
- Place in a freezer bag or container for storing.

Nutritional Value per Serving:

- Calories: around 105.
- Carbohydrates: around 27g.
- Fiber: approximately 3g.
- Protein: around 1g.

Diabetes-Friendly Cake.

Serves: 8

Prep time: 15 minutes.

Cook for 30 minutes.

Ingredients:

- 1 1/2 cups almond flour
- 1/2 cup oat flour.
- One teaspoon of baking powder.
- 3 eggs
- 1/4 cup unsweetened applesauce.
- 1/2 cup erythritol or equivalent sugar alternative.
- 1 teaspoon of vanilla extract.

Instructions:

- Preheat the oven to 350°F/175°C.
- Combine the dry ingredients in one bowl and the liquids in another.
- Combine both ingredients and pour into a greased cake pan.
- Bake for 30 minutes, or until a toothpick comes out clean.

Nutritional Value per Serving:

- Calories: around 200.
- Carbohydrates: around 10g.
- Fiber: approximately 3g.
- Protein: around 6g.

Fruity Ice Cream.

Servings: four.

Preparation time: 10 minutes (including freezing time)

Ingredients:

- Two cups frozen mixed berries.
- One cup of low-fat Greek yogurt
- 2 tablespoons honey (or sugar alternative)

Instructions:

- In a food processor, combine the frozen berries, yogurt, and honey until smooth.
- Transfer to a container and freeze until solid.
- Serve with a spoon or scoop.

Nutritional Value per Serving:

- Calories: around 120.
- Carbohydrates: around 17g.
- Fiber: approximately 2g.
- Protein: around 8g.

Peanut Butter and Jelly Twist

Servings: four.

Prep time: 5 minutes.

Ingredients:

- 4 tablespoons of smooth peanut butter.
- Two tablespoons of low-sugar jelly
- Four slices of low-carb bread

Instructions:

- Spread peanut butter onto two slices of bread.
- Spread jelly on the remaining two pieces.
- Press the slices together to form two sandwiches.
- Divide into strips or creative shapes.

Nutritional Value per Serving:

- Calories: around 200.
- Carbohydrates: around 15g.
- Fiber: approximately 3g.
- Protein: around 8g.

BEVERAGE AND SMOOTHIE RECIPES

Superfood Smoothie

Serves: 1

Prep time: 5 minutes.

Ingredients:

- 1 cup mixed berries (strawberries, raspberries, blueberries)
- One-half ripe avocado
- One cup spinach leaf.
- 1/2 cup of unsweetened almond milk.
- One scoop of protein powder, either vanilla or unflavored.

Instructions:

- Place all items in a blender.
- Blend until smooth.
- Serve immediately.

Nutritional value (estimated):

- Calories: 300.
- Carbohydrate: 20g
- Fiber: 10 grams.
- Protein: 15 grams.

Strawberry Smoothie with Lower Carbs1

Serves: 1

Prep time: 5 minutes.

Ingredients:

- Five medium strawberries.
- One cup of unsweetened soy milk (or almond milk).
- 1/2 cup of low-fat Greek yogurt.
- Six ice cubes

Instructions:

- Combine all ingredients in a blender.
- Blend until smooth.
- Transfer to a glass and garnish with a strawberry.

Nutritional value (estimated):

- Calories: 150.
- Carbohydrates (15g)
- Fiber: 3 grams.
- Protein: 10 grams.

Berry Blast Smoothie

Serves: 1

Prep time: 5 minutes.

Ingredients:

- 1 cup mixed berries, or simply strawberries
- One-quarter handful of baby spinach
- One cup of coconut milk.
- One scoop of vanilla protein.

Instructions:

- Combine all of the ingredients and blend until smooth.
- Indulge instantly.

Nutritional value (estimated):

- Calories: 250.
- Carbohydrates (15g)
- Fiber: 4 grams.
- Protein: 20 grams

Peach Smoothie

Serves: 1

Prep time: 5 minutes.

Ingredients:

- 1/2 cup canned sliced peaches with no sugar added.
- Two tablespoons of non-fat milk.
- 1/2 tablespoon of pure maple syrup or honey.

Instructions:

- Combine all ingredients in a blender.
- Puree until smooth and creamy.
- Store any leftovers in the refrigerator.

Nutritional value (estimated):

- Calories: 100.
- Carbohydrate: 20g
- Fiber: 2 grams.
- Protein: 2 grams

Melon Green Smoothie

Serves: 1

Prep time: 5 minutes.

Ingredients:

- 1 cup of assorted melon balls (cantaloupe, honeydew, or watermelon).
- 1/2 bunch of baby spinach.
- Juice from 1/2 lime.

Instructions:

- In a blender, mix the melon balls, baby spinach, and lime juice.
- Blend until smooth and thoroughly incorporated.
- Pour into a glass and serve immediately.

Nutritional value (estimated):

- Calories: 60.
- Carbohydrates (15g)
- Fiber: 2 grams.
- Protein: 1 gram.

Chocolate Dream Smoothie.

Serves: 1

Prep time: 5 minutes.

Ingredients:

- One-half frozen banana.
- One-quarter cup frozen zucchini
- One-quarter cup frozen avocado
- One handful of baby spinach.
- One tablespoon of almond butter.
- One cup of almond milk.
- One scoop of chocolate protein powder.

Instructions:

- Combine all ingredients in a blender.
- Blend until smooth.
- Serve immediately.

Nutritional value (estimated):

- Calories: 300.
- Carbohydrate: 20g
- Fiber: 6 grams.
- Protein: 15g.

Berry Nut Milkshake

Serves: 1

Prep time: 5 minutes.

Ingredients:

- 1/2 cup mixed berries (including blueberries, strawberries, and raspberries)
- 1/2 cup of unsweetened almond milk.
- 1 tablespoon nut butter of your choice
- 1/2 cup of low-fat Greek yogurt

Instructions:

- Place all items in a blender.
- Blend until smooth.
- Serve cold.

Nutritional value (estimated):

- Calories: 250.
- Carbohydrate: 18g
- Fiber: 4 grams.
- Protein: 10g.

Sweet Potato Kefir Smoothie

Serves: 1

Preparation time: 10 minutes (plus time to prepare sweet potato).

Ingredients:

- 1/2 cooked sweet potato (cooled)
- One cup kefir.
- 1/2 teaspoon cinnamon.
- 1 tablespoon honey (or sugar alternative)

Instructions:

- Steam the sweet potatoes until soft, then cool.
- Combine the sweet potato, kefir, cinnamon, and honey in a blender.
- Blend until smooth.
- Serve cold.

Nutritional value (estimated):

- Calories: 200.
- Carbohydrate: 30g
- Fiber: 5 grams.
- Protein: 8g

Carrot Cake Smoothie

Serves: 1

Prep time: 5 minutes.

Ingredients:

- One tiny carrot, peeled and sliced
- Half cup plain Greek yogurt.
- 1/4 teaspoon turmeric.
- One scoop of unflavored protein powder.
- Half-cup water or almond milk

Instructions:

- Combine all ingredients in a blender.
- Blend until smooth.
- Serve immediately.

Nutritional value (estimated):

- Calories: 150.
- Carbohydrates (15g)
- Fiber: 3 grams.
- Protein: 20g.

Healthy Chocolate Frosty Smoothie.

Serves: 1

Prep time: 5 minutes.

Ingredients:

- One cup unsweetened almond milk.
- One frozen banana.
- One tablespoon of cacao powder
- 1/2 tablespoon cocoa nibs (optional for crunch)
- 1/2 teaspoon vanilla extract.
- 3–5 ice cubes (modify to desired consistency)

Instructions:

- Place all items in a blender.
- Blend until smooth and creamy.
- Serve immediately.

Nutritional value (estimated):

- Calories: 200.
- Carbohydrate: 30g
- Fiber: 6 grams.
- Protein: 5 grams.

CHAPTER 4: BONUS

30 Day Meal Plan

Week 1

Day 1:

- Breakfast: Blueberry smoothie.
- Lunch: Vegetable soup.
- Dinner: Baked chicken and garlic mashed potatoes.
- Snack: plantain chips.
- Beverage: Superfood smoothie.

Day 2:

- Breakfast: Vegetable Omelet.
- Lunch: turkey sandwich.
- Dinner is Spinach and Cheese Stuffed Chicken.
- Snack: Sweet potato chips.
- Beverage: Low-Carb Strawberry Smoothie

Day 3:

- Breakfast: Pumpkin bisque.
- Lunch: Chicken and Goat Cheese Skillet.
- Dinner: Fruit Cocktail.
- Snack: Peanut Butter balls.
- Drink: Berry Blast Smoothie.

Day 4:

- Breakfast: egg muffins.
- Lunch: Curry Chicken Skillet.
- Dinner: Cilantro Bean Burgers.
- Snack: roasted chickpeas.
- Beverage: Peach smoothie.

Day 5:

- Breakfast: Cottage Cheese and Berries
- Lunch: Pressure Cooker Pork Tacos
- Dinner: Egg and Broccoli Slaw Wrap.
- Snack: Hummus
- Drink: Melon Green Smoothie.

Day 6:

- Breakfast: Hard-boiled eggs with avocado.
- Lunch: Chicken with Peach and Avocado Salsa.
- Dinner: Chicken with Low-Fat Crackers
- Snack: Guacamole
- Beverage: Chocolate Dream Smoothie.

Day 7:

- Breakfast: Low Fiber Cereal
- Lunch: Shrimp 'n' Pasta
- Dinner: Vegetable juice.
- Snack: frozen bananas.
- Drink: Berry Nut Milkshake.

Week 2

Day 8:

- Breakfast: Banana smoothie.
- Lunch: Tuna Teriyaki Kabobs.
- Dinner: Fruit purees.
- Snack: Diabetic Friendly Cake
- Drink: Sweet potato kefir smoothie.

Day 9:

- Breakfast: Apple slices with nut butter.
- Lunch: applesauce.
- Dinner is garlic mashed potatoes.
- Snack: Fruit Ice Cream.
- Beverage: carrot cake smoothie.

Day 10:

- Breakfast: Cottage Cheese with Salted Almonds
- Lunch: Milkshake.
- Dinner: baked fish.
- Snack: Peanut butter and jelly twist.
- Drink: Healthy Chocolate Frosty Smoothie.

Week 3

Day 11:

- Breakfast: Apple slices with nut butter.
- Lunch: applesauce.
- Dinner is garlic mashed potatoes.
- Snack: Fruit Ice Cream.
- Beverage: carrot cake smoothie.

Day 12:

- Breakfast: Cottage Cheese with Salted Almonds
- Lunch: Milkshake.
- Dinner: baked fish.
- Snack: Peanut butter and jelly twist.
- Drink: Healthy Chocolate Frosty Smoothie.

Day 13:

- Breakfast: Blueberry smoothie.
- Lunch: Vegetable soup.
- Dinner is Spinach and Cheese Stuffed Chicken.
- Snack: Sweet potato chips.
- Beverage: Low-Carb Strawberry Smoothie

Day 14:

- Breakfast: Pumpkin bisque.
- Lunch: Chicken and Goat Cheese Skillet.
- Dinner: Fruit Cocktail.
- Snack: Peanut Butter balls.
- Drink: Berry Blast Smoothie.

Day 15:

- Breakfast: egg muffins.
- Lunch: Curry Chicken Skillet.
- Dinner: Cilantro Bean Burgers.
- Snack: roasted chickpeas.
- Beverage: Peach smoothie.

Day 16:

- Breakfast: Cottage Cheese and Berries
- Lunch: Pressure Cooker Pork Tacos
- Dinner: Egg and Broccoli Slaw Wrap.
- Snack: Hummus
- Drink: Melon Green Smoothie.

Day 17:

- Breakfast: Hard-boiled eggs with avocado.
- Lunch: Chicken with Peach and Avocado Salsa.
- Dinner: Chicken with Low-Fat Crackers
- Snack: Guacamole
- Beverage: Chocolate Dream Smoothie.

Week 4

Day 18:

- Breakfast: Low Fiber Cereal
- Lunch: Shrimp 'n' Pasta
- Dinner: Vegetable juice.
- Snack: frozen bananas.
- Drink: Berry Nut Milkshake.

Day 19:

- Breakfast: Banana smoothie.
- Lunch: Tuna Teriyaki Kabobs.
- Dinner: applesauce.
- Snack: Diabetic Friendly Cake
- Drink: Fruity Ice Cream.

Day 20:

- Breakfast: Apple slices with nut butter.
- Lunch: Chicken with Peach and Avocado Salsa.
- Dinner: Chicken with Low-Fat Crackers
- Snack: Guacamole
- Beverage: Chocolate Dream Smoothie.

Day 21:

- Breakfast: Cottage Cheese with Salted Almonds
- Lunch: Milkshake.
- Dinner: baked fish.

- Snack: Peanut butter and jelly twist.
- Drink: Healthy Chocolate Frosty Smoothie.

Day 22:

- Breakfast: Blueberry smoothie.
- Lunch: Vegetable soup.
- Dinner is Spinach and Cheese Stuffed Chicken.
- Snack: Sweet potato chips.
- Beverage: Low-Carb Strawberry Smoothie

Day 23:

- Breakfast: Pumpkin bisque.
- Lunch: Chicken and Goat Cheese Skillet.
- Dinner: Fruit Cocktail.
- Snack: Peanut Butter balls.
- Drink: Berry Blast Smoothie.

Day 24:

- Breakfast: egg muffins.
- Lunch: Curry Chicken Skillet.
- Dinner: Cilantro Bean Burgers.
- Snack: roasted chickpeas.
- Beverage: Peach smoothie.

Week 5

Day 25:

- Breakfast: Apple slices with nut butter.
- Lunch: Chicken and Low-Fat Crackers
- Dinner: Vegetable soup.
- Snack: Guacamole
- Beverage: Chocolate Dream Smoothie.

Day 26:

- Breakfast: Low Fiber Cereal
- Lunch: Shrimp 'n' Pasta
- Dinner: Vegetable juice.
- Snack: frozen bananas.
- Drink: Berry Nut Milkshake.

Day 27:

- Breakfast: Banana smoothie.
- Lunch: Tuna Teriyaki Kabobs.
- Dinner: applesauce.
- Snack: Diabetic Friendly Cake
- Drink: Fruity Ice Cream.

Day 28:

- Breakfast: Apple slices with nut butter.
- Lunch: Chicken with Peach and Avocado Salsa.
- Dinner is garlic mashed potatoes.
- Snack: Peanut butter and jelly twist.
- Drink: Healthy Chocolate Frosty Smoothie.

Day 29:

- Breakfast: Cottage Cheese with Salted Almonds
- Lunch: Milkshake.
- Dinner: baked fish.
- Snack: roasted chickpeas.
- Beverage: Peach smoothie.

Day 30:

- Breakfast: Hard-boiled eggs with avocado.
- Lunch: Vegetable soup.
- Dinner is Spinach and Cheese Stuffed Chicken.
- Snack: Sweet potato chips.
- Beverage: Low-Carb Strawberry Smoothie

Grocery Shopping List for Diabetic Gastroparesis

Fruits:

- Ripe bananas.
- Berries: strawberries, blueberries, raspberries.
- Melon (Cantaloupe, Honeydew)
- Canned or cooked fruit (applesauce, peaches, pears)

Vegetables:

- Cooked or canned veggies (such as carrots, zucchini, squash, and green beans).
- Vegetable juice (low sodium).
- Avocado (ripe)

Grains and Starches:

Bread:

- White bread.
- English Muffins
- Plain bagels.
- Low-fiber tortillas

Cereals:

- Cream of Wheat.
- Rice Krispies.
- Instant oatmeal (plain).
- Cornflakes.

Other:

- White rice.
- Refined pasta.
- Low sodium crackers

Protein:

- Eggs, prepared in various ways.

Lean Proteins:

- Ground chicken or turkey.
- Fish (whitefish, salmon, and tilapia).
- Tofu
- Fully cooked beans (lentils, black beans, pinto beans)

Nut Butters:

- Smooth peanut butter (natural)
- Almond butter, smooth and natural
- Smooth, all-natural cashew butter

Dairy and Alternatives:

Milk:

- Low-fat or skim milk.
- Lactose-free milk.
- Plant milk (unsweetened almond, rice, or soy milk)

Yogurt:

- Yogurt with low or no fat (simple or Greek)
- Dairy-free, unsweetened yogurt

Cheese:

- Cottage Cheese.
- Cream Cheese
- Mild cheddar cheese.

Other:

- The broth:
- Low-sodium chicken or veggie broth.

Oils:

- Olive Oil.
- Avocado oil.

Condiments:

- Herbs, spices
- Lemon Juice
- Vinegar (balsamic or apple cider).

Sweeteners:

- Stevia
- Monkey fruit
- Use little amounts of honey or maple syrup (see your doctor).

Tips For Using This List:

- Read the labels: Look for low-fiber, low-fat, and low-sugar products.
- Fresh vs. Frozen/Canned: While fresh is preferable, frozen or canned veggies and fruits can be a practical substitute. Search for "no sugar added" choices.
- Cook thoroughly: All vegetables should be cooked till soft for ease digestion.
- Portion Control: Even with permitted foods, moderation is essential.
- Consult Your Doctor: Always consult with your doctor or dietician for specialized advice on your individual needs and constraints.

Additional Considerations:

- Hydration: Water is essential for gastroparesis. Add herbal teas and clear broths to your grocery list.
- Variety: To establish a balanced diet, eat a variety of foods from each category.
- Listen to Your Body: Pay attention to how your body reacts to different foods and make adjustments accordingly.

This list is a beginning point. Customize it to reflect your preferences and any dietary limitations you may have. Remember, effective diabetic gastroparesis management requires close collaboration with a healthcare practitioner.

Tips for Dining Out and Social Gatherings

Eating out and attending social gatherings might be difficult when you have diabetic gastroparesis, but with the appropriate methods, you can still have fun. Here are some suggestions to assist you handle dining out and social gatherings:

Eating out.

- Plan Ahead: Before you travel, review the restaurant's menu online to find gastroparesis-friendly options1.
- Communicate Your Needs: Don't be afraid to ask the server about ingredients or request changes to dishes if necessary.
- Eat Slowly: Chew your food completely to promote digestion and avoid discomfort.
- Portion Control: To prevent exacerbating gastroparesis symptoms, order an appetizer as your main course or share a dish.
- Avoid Trigger diets: High-fat, fried, and fiber-rich diets can impede gastric emptying.
- Maintain an upright posture for at least an hour after eating to help digestion.

Social Gatherings

- Bring Your Own Food: If you're not sure about the menu, bring a gastroparesis-friendly item to eat.

- Inform the Host: Let the host know about your dietary limitations so that they can meet your demands.
- Prioritize socializing: Instead, then focusing on food, enjoy the company of friends and family.
- Keep an eye on your blood sugar levels, especially if your meal plan is disrupted.
- Limit Alcohol: Alcohol can impact blood sugar levels and gastroparesis symptoms, therefore limit or avoid it.
- Stay Active: After eating, gentle walking can aid digestion and blood sugar regulation.

Remember, these are basic guidelines that may need to be modified based on your specific experiences and dietary preferences. Consult your healthcare provider for specific guidance.

CONCLUSION

As we reach the last page of "Diabetic Gastroparesis Diet Cookbook," I hope you feel a sense of achievement and empowerment. This book was written not just to educate you through the culinary aspects of controlling diabetic gastroparesis, but also to instill confidence in your nutritional choices and inventiveness in the kitchen.

You now have a vital tool that allows you to regulate your health through informed food choices. Each dish was designed with your specific needs in mind, combining nutrients with the enjoyment of eating.

I am really glad for the opportunity to share this collection of recipes with you. Your health journey is unique and ongoing; therefore, I encourage you to keep exploring the Flavors and possibilities that each dish provides. Remember that each meal provides an opportunity to fuel your body while also bringing joy into your day.

As you embark on this gastronomic journey, I invite you to share your thoughts. Your candid reviews and positive feedback are not only greatly appreciated, but also serve as a beacon for others embarking on their own journeys with diabetic gastroparesis. Please take a moment to share your comments and tell us how this cookbook has impacted your life.

Managing diabetic gastroparesis is an ongoing and personal struggle. Stay curious, flexible, and, most importantly, aware of your body's demands. Your opinions, stories, and insights are vital as we continue to learn and grow as a community.

May your kitchen be filled with delectable scents, your plates with nutritious food, and your heart full of contentment. **Here's to many more dinners honoring health, happiness, and the simple pleasures of eating well.**

Made in the USA
Las Vegas, NV
15 October 2024